Ultimate Dash Diet Smoothie Guide

AMARPREET SINGH

Publisher - The Thought Flame

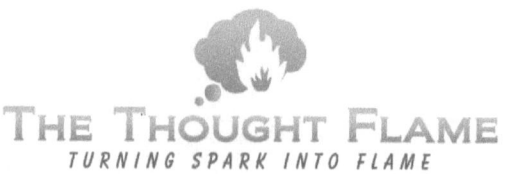

info@thethoughtflame.com

www.thethoughtflame.com

Table of Contents

Introduction

With an estimated seven out of ten Americans now taking at least one prescription drug, the emphasis on achieving good health is now stronger than it has ever been.

Ranked as one of the healthiest diets, and the best diet for diabetes four years in a row, the DASH diet has been hailed as 'the diet for all diseases', and has been proven to improve health over a variety of conditions.

The DASH diet stands for 'Dietary Approaches to Stop Hypertension'. It was originally developed by the US National Institute of Health, as a way to lower blood pressure without medication.

By following the dietary advice within the DASH diet, it is possible to reduce your blood pressure by a few points in as little as two weeks. Prolonged use of the diet can see systolic blood pressure reduced by as much as 12 points, which is significant in treating high blood pressure and its resultant effects.

Lowered risk of heart disease, stroke, cholesterol, kidney failure, and several types of cancer, are all benefits of the DASH diet. More so, with its emphasis on real foods, especially fruits and vegetables, and the right amount of protein, the DASH diet has proven itself to be a great weight loss tool.

In this book you will find proven weight loss ideas and Dash Diet smoothie recipes that will help you meet your health and weight loss goals. Come try the diet that thousands of others have already had incredible success with and begin to get healthy and lose weight.

Chapter One: What Is The Dash Diet and What Does It Entail?

It is quite alarming that the number of people suffering from high blood pressure is increasing with each passing day. While high blood pressure may be accelerated by a high salt diet, salt is not the only thing that may cause blood pressure. If you are obese or overweight, you also have a higher chance of having high blood pressure. Other causes of high blood pressure include stress, too much alcohol consumption, old age, genetics and chronic kidney disease as well as other types of adrenal and thyroid disorders.

You may probably be wondering so where does DASH diet come into play. DASH simply stands for Dietary Approaches to Stop

Hypertension. This is mainly because the main causes of Hypertension are usually closely related with your diet. Therefore, if you have hypertension, the best way to address the issues is to change your diet rather than rely on pills only. The DASH diet has actually been shown to lower blood pressure within as little as 14 days. Can you imagine this?

What Does This Diet Entail?

This diet plan mainly focuses on consumption of whole grains, nuts, fish, poultry and low fat diet. When on this diet, you consume less of sugar, red meat, fat and sugary drinks. The DASH diet is usually recommended for people with high blood pressure since it meets the low-sodium requirements that are suitable for those suffering from hypertension.

Chapter Two: Specific Guidelines For The Dash Diet

The DASH diet is an eating plan that is high in potassium, magnesium, and calcium. It is low in sodium, rich in fruits and vegetables, and low in fat or non-fat dairy.

Grains, especially whole grains, lean meat, fish, poultry, and nuts and beans make up the rest of the diet. High in fiber and low in fat, it is a healthier way of eating, flexible enough to adapt to the lifestyles of most people.

Here the following guidelines for this diet:

-Fiber is 30 grams

-Carbohydrates are 55% calories

-Cholesterol is limited to 150 milligrams

-Protein is 18% calories

-Saturated Fat is 65% calories

-Fiber is 30grams

-Total Fat is 27% calories

I know that this can all be kind of confusing so I will break it down further for you so it is easier to understand.

Grain Products and Grains

-These include English muffins, bagels, cereals, grits, whole wheat bread, oatmeal, unsalted pretzels, crackers and popcorn.

-The required serving size is 7-8 servings.

-An example of such a serving includes: 1 slice of bread, 1 oz dry cereal and ½ cup cooked rice, cereal or pasta.

-Since your goal is not to lower blood pressure but to lose weight, you can reduce your carbohydrate intake to 4 to 5 servings.

Fruits

-4-5 daily servings of fruits are enough. Some common fruits to take when on a dash diet include grapes, dates, mangoes, tangerines, grapefruit, banana , pineapple , apple, melon, kiwi, avocado, berries and oranges among many other fruits.

-A suitable daily serving will be 1 medium fruit, ¼-cup dried fruit, ½-cup fresh fruit and 6 oz. fresh fruit juice.

Dry Beans, Seeds and Nuts

-Some of these include mixed nuts, walnuts, peanuts, sunflower seeds, lentils, kidney beans, peas and lentils. You are only required to take around 4-5 servings of dry beans, seeds and nuts each week. Nuts can be quite high in salt so try to look for unsalted nuts.

Sugars and Sweets

-You need to try to keep your intake of things like maple syrup, jelly, sugar, fruit-flavored gelatin, hard candy, ices, fruit punch, sorbet, jellybeans and jam. If you need to take sweets, ensure that they are low in fats.

Vegetables

-Vegetables are usually important since they are rich in fiber, magnesium and potassium.

-Some common vegetables you can take include potatoes, carrots, green peas, broccoli, squash, spinach, kales, collards, green beans, artichokes, sweet potatoes, lima beans, turnip greens and tomatoes.

-The appropriate vegetable serving is 4-5 servings. However, since you have reduced your intake of carbohydrates, you can increase your serving to 5-6 servings.

-An example of 4-5 servings include: ½ cup cooked vegetables, 6 ounce vegetable juice and 1 cup raw leafy vegetables.

Meat, Poultry and Fish

-Meat is an amazing source of magnesium and protein. The recommended serving of meat is 2 or less servings, which is around 3 oz. cooked meat, fish or poultry.

Fat Free or Low Fat Dairy

-Dairy products are usually very important, as they are major sources of protein and calcium.

-The most appropriate serving when on a dash diet is 2-3 servings.

-An example of such a serving is 1 cup yogurt, 8 oz. milk, and 1 ½ oz cheese.

Fats and Oils

-2-3 servings of fats and oils daily is just enough. Ensure that you are consuming trans - fat free fats and oils. You do not want to consume more fat and yet you are trying to burn fat. This may however vary depending on the amount of carbohydrates you consume. For instance, if you take fewer carbohydrates, you would want to increase your intake of fats and oils to ensure that your metabolism does not slow down and you still have enough energy.

-Suitable serving sizes include 1-teaspoon soft margarine, 1-tablespoon low fat mayonnaise, 1-teaspoon vegetable oil and 2 tablespoons light salad dressing.

Chapter Three: How The Dash Diet Will Help You To Lose Weight

I am sure you are probably wondering 'if the DASH diet is suitable for people who are looking to lower their blood pressure, where do I come in when I want to adopt the diet to lose weight. You will be glad to know that the DASH diet is very relevant if you would want to lose weight. This is mainly because the diet focuses on reduction of intake of sugary foods, processed foods and high carbohydrate foods, which all eventually lead to weight gain. The diet instead focuses on consumption of more fruits, vegetables, healthy fats and more of whole foods.

So how do you lose weight with the DASH Diet? The dash diet enables you to eat more of fruits, vegetables and whole foods that are quite satisfying . What this means is that you will feel hungry less often and thus reducing the number of times you eat throughout the day since you are full. Furthermore, the diet also focuses on consuming a high amount of dairy products that are high in calcium and we all know that calcium rich products favor weight loss.

This is mainly since calcium stored in the fat cells usually determines how fat is broken down and stored by the body. This simply means that the more calcium in a fat cell, the more fat it will burn. This is why the meal plan focused greatly on consumption of dairy products. The key is however not to just take any dairy products but rather to take dairy products that are fat-free or low in fat.

Why Does The Dash Diet Help For Weight Loss

With there being many diets, you may be wondering which diet to choose. The DASH diet has been shown to be very effective for weight loss due to a number of things even though it was not initially started to achieve weight loss . Most diets usually do not work owing to the high calorie deficit.

This is however not the case with this diet. The DASH diet allows you to eat all food groups but in moderation. When you think of all the fad diets that promise fast weight loss, it is usually very hard for you to stick to such a diet. For instance, some people may recommend the consumption of smoothies, juices and a no carb diet in order to lose weight. While you may lose weight, quickly, you are likely to gain it all back again.

DASH diet is not a fad diet but rather a lifestyle diet . Considering that this diet is suitable for people with hypertension, such people need to consume this diet to maintain their blood pressure. You can thus be sure that by adopting this diet, you will not only lose weight but also reduce your risk of getting heart attack, heart failure, stroke and other heart diseases.

Chapter Four: Why Smoothies and What Are Their Benefits?

Smoothies are blended drinks made predominately with fruits. However, they can also be made with leafy green vegetables. You can also add dairy milk, nut milks, peanut butte, r and yogurts to smoothies.

What Are The Benefits of Smoothies?

There are many health benefits to drinking smoothies and you can expect to experience at least some of these:

1. Improved Hydration

Smoothies are full of water, from the fruits and veggies to the dairy products, which are largely water. Drinking a smoothie for breakfast is a good way to ensure that you start the day fully hydrated.

Increased energy, focus and mental clarity – increasing your intake for fruits and vegetables will leave you with bags of energy. In turn, this will lead to increased focus and mental clarity. No more brain fog!

2. A Much Better Immune System

Eating a diet that is full of essential nutrients, vitamins and anti-oxidants, ensures our immune systems are working to the best of their ability. You can expect less colds, bugs and infections when eating this way.

3. Getting A Better Nights Sleep

A body that is well hydrated and full of the right nutrition, functions in a better way. This includes sleep.

4. Improve Your Digestive System

Eating a natural diet that is full of fruits, vegetables and fiber, means that our digestive systems work better, and our bowel movements become more regular.

5. Releases Toxins From Your Body

Giving the body good nutrition, in an easily assailable form , such as liquids, allows it time to 'clean house' and release toxins that have built up over time.

Why Dash Diet Smoothies Are Good For You

Many smoothies on the market today are made from fruit concentrates, syrups and added sugars, preservatives and flavorings.

DASH smoothies are made from fresh fruits and vegetables and contain no added sugars. Fresh is definitely best, and with a DASH smoothie you are guaranteed of getting all the goodness with none of the nasties.

Chapter Five: How To Get Started On The Dash Diet

You have finally done it! You have finally taken the initiative to better yourself. You know that one of the biggest things that you have to do is to work on your health. After all, better health means a better you. You have done all the research that is available to you about the Dash diet and you have decided that it is time to get started. That is the exact moment that you stop and wonder how in the world do I get started?

Have Motivation and Commitment

Getting started is easier than you think. The very first thing you have to do is commit to the idea. This is the most important part of the whole 'better you' process. A diet is only as efficient as the dieter's will to succeed; so unless you are ready to fully commit to the idea, you will not be ready to get started. Motivation is the best friend to commitment.

You can use different motivators such as an awesome new dress or an expensive pair of feel-good shoes to motivate yourself to do almost anything. Motivation is another key to successful dieting.

Plan A Trip To The Doctor's Office

It is time to head to your friendly neighborhood doctor. This is such an important step that a lot of people skip. Unless you have a degree in biology, chemistry , or nutrition you probably have no real idea how your body runs and the appropriate amounts of nutrition needed to sustain wellness. This is where your doctor comes in. A doctor can take in all the information that you have gathered and help you to formulate the best exercise and eating plans so that you can lose weight without risking harm to yourself. It is also important to go consult with a doctor in the event that you have a disease or a family history of diseases such as high blood pressure , diabetes, or heart disease, in order to be monitored more specifically. Who knows, maybe your results will help your doctor prescribe the Dash diet to someone else in need.

Prepare Your Home For Your New Diet

Once you have obtained your doctor's blessing it is important to go through your house and get rid of all the processed fatty foods that will tempt you to stray from dieting. You don't have to throw them away, but you need to get them out of your eyesight. Go around your neighborhood or to less privileged neighborhoods and donate the boxes of extra food to people in need. They will appreciate the food and it will allow you to start your diet with a clean slate. Yes, this means all of your secret stashes of snacks have got to go. Don't try to deny that you have a secret stash of snacks; we all do and we all secretly eat chocolates in the corner while no one is looking.

This is a great time to put your research skills to work. You need to start looking for awesome recipes that will help you make healthy meals without having to sacrifice taste. It is also a good idea to locate some local farms or farmer markets that will be able to provide fresher produce choices. If the area you live in does not have these options that is fine. Most of the supermarkets have everything that you need to maintain your dietary guidelines. Just always be conscious of labels, and make sure that you always keep an eye on the sugar and sodium levels of every piece of food that you pick up to take home with you.

Exercise Frequently

Now here is the hard part, you have to exercise. There is no such thing as a miracle diet that can help you reach your goal weight without a little extra work put into it. If there was then everyone would be skinny.

Exercising does not have to be evil . If you think of exercising as every time you move, instead of sectioning off certain things like walking twenty minutes or running around the track, you will find it much easier. If you need to walk for twenty minutes, go to the store and browse through different areas. Any shopper knows that at large supermarkets you walk everywhere, and half the time you have to go across the store half a dozen times because you forgot something.

You can vary the speed in which you walk. If you have problems with being able to deny yourself, steer clear of the food aisles and instead go through the clothes aisle and pick out a new skinny outfit that you will buy after you hit your target weight. If you are feeling adventurous you can go out to the swimming pool or go out for a brisk run in the park. Bicycling is also a wonderful way to get in the extra exercise that you need and burn lots of calories. You can plan a hike in the woods with friends to help keep you motivated. There are a million other ways to exercise, you just have to find the right one that works for you.

If you are having a rough day, clean something. It is exercise: sweeping or mopping floors or stretching up high to get that dust off the fan blades. If that does not work, go to the store and purchase a new work out outfit. You will immediately feel better about working out if you have an appealing outfit and a comfortable pair of shoes to wear.

Chapter Six: Healthy Dash Diet Smoothie Recipes

All you need to make smoothies is a blender, or a smoothie maker. If you use a blender, make sure it has a 2-3 liter jug on it. Note, the higher the speed of your blender, the easier it will be to completely blend your smoothies.

Simply make sure you have a good variety of fruits , milk and leafy green vegetables to hand. Try to buy organic produce where possible as the aim with a healthier diet is to put as much good into the body as we can.

Peach and Orange Smoothie

With the tangy flavor or oranges and the sweet flavor of peaches, this is one smoothie recipe that will give you the extra energy boost that you are looking for.

Makes: 2 Glasses

Ingredients:

-1 Cup of Orange Juice, Freshly Squeezed

-1 Orange, Large In Size or 2 Oranges, Small In Size

-1 Peach, De-Stoned and Sliced Into Fine Slices

-1 Mango, Peeled and Cut Into Thin Slices

Directions:

1. Add all of your ingredients into your blender and blend until smooth in consistency. Add in some water if you want a thinner consistency and serve immediately.

Apricot and Orange Smoothie

This is a smoothie that you will love to enjoy during the summer month. Savory and filling, this smoothie recipe will be one that you will want to make and serve every day during the summer.

Makes: 1 Glass

Ingredients:

-1 Cup of Orange Juice, Freshly Squeezed

-½ Cup of Apricots, Tinned In Fruit Juice

-1 Cup of Grapes, White and Seedless

Directions:

1. First drain your apricots and add all of your ingredients into your blender and blend until smooth in consistency. Add any additional water if you want a thinner consistency and serve at once.

Coconut Cream and Banana Smoothie

Even though you are on a diet, that does not mean that you cannot spoil yourself every once in a while. This is the perfect recipe to spoil yourself with and to serve whenever you want to kick back.

Makes: 2 Glasses

Ingredients:

-1 Banana, Large In Size and Frozen

-½ Cup of Romaine Lettuce, Roughly Chopped

-1 Cup of Coconut Water

-¼ Cup of Coconut, Shredded, Dried and Unsweetened

-1 Medjool Date, Finely Chopped

-¼ tsp. of Vanilla Extract

Directions:

1. Place all of your ingredients into your blender and blend until smooth in consistency. Add any additional water if you want your smoothie to be thinner in consistency. Serve after blending and enjoy.

Healthy Cucumber and Blackberry Smoothie

If you are looking for a smoothie recipe that has a much more richer taste than you are accustomed to, then this is the perfect recipe for you. The blackberries add a nice and fresh taste to this recipe, making it one that you will want to enjoy again and again.

Makes: 1 Glass

Ingredients:

-½ Cup of Blackberries, Fresh or Frozen

-½ Of A Banana, Fresh and Large In Size

-½ - 1 Cup of Low Fat Milk or Fat-Free Milk or Almond Milk.

Directions:

1. Place all of your ingredients into a blender and blend until smooth in consistency and serve at once.

Fruity Berry Smoothie

This smoothie recipes is packed full of the different kinds of delicious berries that you will certainly enjoy. Extremely fruity and absolutely delicious, this is one recipe that will leave you wanting more.

Makes: 2 Glass

Ingredients:

-½ Cup of Pineapple, Fresh, Peeled and Finely Chopped

-½ Cup of Blackberries, Fresh

-½ Cup of Blueberries, Fresh

-½ Cup of Low Fat or Fat-Free Yogurt

-½ Cup Low Fat or Fat-Free Milk or Almond Milk

Directions:

1. Add all of your ingredients into a blender and blend until very smooth in consistency. Add in some extra water for a thinner consistency and serve immediately. Enjoy.

Conclusion

It is such a pity that we are an overweight society that is always eating processed foods and foods that are high in sugars. It no wonder that we are seeing very high numbers of people who are obese or overweight. If you need to lose weight, you need to take the right steps to achieve this. Adopting the DASH diet is a great idea considering all the benefits of this diet like not having to starve yourself in order to lose weight. With this diet, you are sure that you will not only lose weight but will also adopt better eating habits that will enable you to live a healthier life.

There is a saying that 'health is wealth,' and it is a statement that is especially true in a society where one in three people suffer from high blood pressure.

Having high blood pressure can not only cause a risk of heart disease, kidney disease and stroke, but it can also increase the chances of developing certain cancers, diabetes, osteoporosis, and many other diseases.

It makes sense that the more we look after our health, the better our chances of not developing any of these potential life threatening diseases becomes.

The DASH diet offers the perfect solution. A food plan that is easy to follow, interesting to eat, and won't leave will feeling like you are constantly on a 'diet'. The great indirect effects of following this eating plan will also see you losing weight! It really is a win-win situation!

Taking the time to incorporate the principles of the DASH diet into your lifestyle, on a permanent basis, is certainly a step worth aiming for.

I hope this book will enable you to make healthier choices to enable you achieve your desired weight loss goals.

About Us

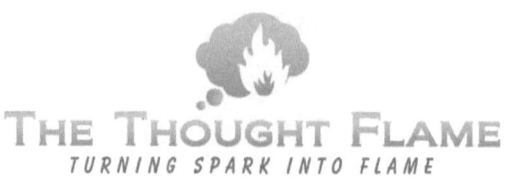

The Thought Flame is committed to add value to its customers through various books, online courses and other resources. You can learn more about us and our books at www.thethoughtflame.com.

Don't forget to check out our amazing **online video courses** at www.thethoughtflame.com/courses/ to take your knowledge to another level.

To check out our **extraordinary collection of diet/cookbooks**, visit http://www.thethoughtflame.com/category/non-fictional/cookbooks/ .

As a part of our valued relationship with our customers, we keep providing you free promotional books, courses and other stuff on subscribing with us on our site. We have a strict anti-spam policy and assure you no spam mails will be sent to your mailbox.

To subscribe with us, visit www.thethoughtflame.com.

Like our work and would like to say thanks? Buy us a cup of coffee at www.thethoughtflame.com/coffee/

Author

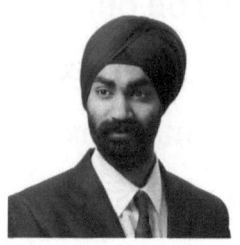

Amarpreet Singh is an avid learner and his passion for education has made him travel, work and study all across the world. He holds three masters degrees, including MBA, from top universities in Asia.

He is author of dozens of books, many of which are Amazon's bestseller, varying in various topics and categories. He also teaches many online courses having thousands of students across the world.

He has a keen interest in international affairs, economics, global poverty and politics, financial markets and entrepreneurship, and strives to be part of a community that shares the same passion.

He has worked as consultant with organizations like Airbus and The World Bank.

He loves travelling and learning about new cultures, and has been fortunate to live/work/travel/study in countries like India, China, Korea, US, South Africa, Japan, Philippines, Singapore, Canada etc., and learn about the culture and lifestyle in each of them.

To check out more of his work, visit

www.thethoughtflame.com